ARTHRITIS
AND
RHEUMATISM

HERBAL REMEDIES

ARTHRITIS AND RHEUMATISM

MERVYN MITTON

Edited by David Potterton ND, MRN, MNIMH
*Consultant Medical Herbalist and
Registered Naturopath*

foulsham

LONDON · NEW YORK · TORONTO · SYDNEY

Preface

In the early years of this century most medicines were based on herbs. Indeed, many remedies prescribed by doctors had been used with success down the centuries. Even as late as the 1940s about half of all prescriptions still contained herbal ingredients.

During the sixties and seventies, the medical profession began to discard the older, proven methods of treatment in favour of newer chemical-based drugs. Although pharmaceutical research has produced life-saving drugs, there have also been unfortunate results due to the over-reliance on drug therapy for less serious ailments. We now frequently hear reports of side effects — some of them serious — from many of these relatively untested medicines. A number of drugs have had to be withdrawn from the market.

Within the last few years, however, there has been a dramatic resurgence of interest, both from the medical profession and the public, in alternative and complementary forms of treatment, of which herbal medicine remains the most popular.

The author of this book, Mr Mitton, was a consulting herbalist at Cathay of Bournemouth, a large retail herbal business established by his parents many years ago.

This revised edition of his book gives relevant information and advice to the seeker of good health who wishes to know more about herbal medicine.

Contents

Introduction

During the Second World War — and even today in some research laboratories and American prisons — human guinea pigs were used to test new drugs and their effect on the human system. The inducements for taking these risks were usually either a payment, or in the case of prisoners, a remission of their sentence.

Unfortunately, no freedom of choice or inducements have been made to the many thousands of unfortunate patients who, over the last few years, have been subjected to an unintentional 'guinea pig' testing of new arthritic and rheumatic drugs, some of which have been obviously launched in advance of a complete knowledge of their safety and which were subsequently suspended by the Committee on the Safety of Medicines.

At least two drugs have been associated with deaths in arthritis patients, with several thousand cases or reported side effects including nausea, dyspepsia, vomiting, haemorrhaging, nail separation, headaches and sun-sensitivity. One caused severe headaches and gastro-intestinal problems, including haemorrhaging.

Another anti-inflammatory drug had its licence revoked. Of about 10,000 patients taking it, 217 were thought to have suffered side effects such as upset stomach, stomach ulcer irritation and internal bleeding, and for some, dizziness and headaches.

Since rheumatoid arthritis and osteoarthritis have such serious and debilitating effects, it is not surprising that so many drugs have been tried over the years to alleviate the symptoms. However, many of these drugs have had side effects and in some cases these have been more serious than the condition for which they were prescribed. In addition to the drugs listed later, must be considered the potentially serious side effects of pain-killers such as distalgesic, paracetamol and aspirin.

Before I am accused of attacking the pharmaceutical industry indiscriminately, I would like to point out that there are many alternative herbal tablets and infusions which can be used for the same anti-inflammatory purposes but with few, if any, of the side-effects. Herbal medicine has never been in opposition to the medical profession, but is rather the original and alternative method of treating illness by natural means. With the side effects possible from some of the chemical drugs, I believe it is sensible to look at safer alternatives first, before taking potentially serious risks.

It is obvious that there is a need for help and advice for everyone troubled by rheumatism and arthritis — and that this should be based on the known properties of herbs is equally reasonable, since in many cases they can be easily prepared or taken at home. Home treatment has a place, since experience shows that many people prefer to try to control their problem themselves before seeking professional help.

This does not imply that where a serious medical condition exists it should be treated at home from the advice given in this book. In such a case, one should always contact a physician or medical herbalist. However, where the pattern of the problem matches examples given, and where the advice is applicable, then herbal treatment could well be the answer.

Words of Caution

Herbal medicines are generally safe, but they are not without their contraindications. Therefore:

1 Never take any herbal medication during pregnancy without advice from a qualified practitioner.

2 Do not treat babies and young children, or the very elderly without obtaining professional advice as dosages are much more critical.

3 Do not take herbal medicines if you are also taking medicines from your own doctor, as the two may interact. Do not stop taking medicines prescribed by a doctor without advice.

4 Do not self treat if you are suffering from a liver condition or heart disease.

5 Always use herbs from reputable suppliers, preferably from a medical herbalist. Do not gather medicinal plants from the wild.

Note: Because it is recognised that there are contra-indications and that individuals may react differently to herbal remedies, the author and publishers emphasise that they cannot be held liable for any adverse effects caused by self-treatment with any of the remedies mentioned in this book. Self-treatment must be undertaken according to the individual's own judgement.

Chapter 1

Identifying Your Illness

It is likely that most people suffering from a rheumatic or arthritic condition will have already sought medical advice and have had a correct diagnosis made. However, sometimes complications arise, or the condition is not thought serious enough to worry the doctor, and it is for this reason that a description of the various illnesses and their symptoms is given.

Many readers will be dedicated already to the use of natural medicines; others may have tried alternative treatments without success. The most important thing is to ensure that you have correctly identified your condition before commencing the treatments outlined here as a misdiagnosis could lead to a deterioration in your health.

Second, remember that herbal treatment is relatively slow-acting and generally relies on a gradual build-up in the system. This makes it particularly suitable for long-term arthritic and rheumatic complaints since herbs are usually without side-effects, not addictive and are compatible with one another.

RHEUMATISM

This is an umbrella term applied to diseases which have inflammation or degenerative action on the muscles, joints and other parts of the body. The various forms of this illness can usually be summarised as follows:

ACUTE RHEUMATISM
More usually known as rheumatic fever, this is now a rare disease. This condition requires specialist medical treatment.

NON-ARTICULAR RHEUMATISM
A number of common illnesses come under this category. They are often known as muscular rheumatism. Most have a tendency to become worse in cold, damp weather and to show improvement when it is warmer.

Many herbs have been found to be of benefit for these conditions. Also the application of gentle heat can bring comfort together with mild exercise and warm clothing.

ASSOCIATED CONDITIONS

Some conditions associated with rheumatism are described below.

BURSITIS
These are inflammations within the 'pocket' areas in the body at points where there is a lot of movement. They are most common at elbows, knees and also at the shoulder, giving rise to the painful 'frozen shoulder'. Housemaid's knee and tennis elbow are two common names given when the inflammation is localised. Massage with a good rheumatic balm will often give relief.

FIBROSITIS
This is another form of muscular rheumatism, particularly when inflammation puts pressure on the endings of the sensory nerves.

LUMBAGO
A form of low back pain, lumbago is usually seated in the

muscles, particularly when they have been subjected to strain or damage. Sometimes linked with rheumatic attacks in other parts of the body, lumbago often has pain of a sharp stabbing type and can be very incapacitating.

MYALGIA
This is a medical term used to describe muscular pain. Rheumatic polymyalgia occurs almost exclusively in the elderly in which there is severe aching and stiffness of the neck, the upper arms and shoulders and of the pelvic area and thighs.

NEURITIS
An inflammation of the nerves, this can be of a restrictive nature as with sciatica attacks.

SCIATICA
A common complaint, sufferers of sciatica usually have it as a result of a prolapsed intervertebral disc pressing on the sciatic nerve. The pain runs down the sciatic nerve through the buttocks into the back of the leg and sometimes into the foot — the side affected depends on where the pressure from the disc is being applied.

GOUT

In the past, sufferers of gout were figures of fun — perhaps because it was associated with good living, and, therefore, in less affluent times, was felt to be deserved.

More prone to attack those above middle years, gout is an acute and chronic inflammatory arthritis caused by an excess of uric acid in the system, which can lay down deposits of sodium urate in the joints. High living in the form of rich food and too much alcohol can be contributory factors. Gout can be hereditary.

Symptoms of an attack can include stomach upsets, liver and sometimes bladder disturbance and excruciating pain — often in the ball of the great toe, but sometimes in the heel or thumb. The affected part swells and takes on a deep red colour. The pain may subside after a few hours, but the normal pattern is for it to return nightly for a week to ten days — the usual period of an attack.

Gout is one of the most painful conditions dealt with in this book and being of a degenerative nature, always presents problems.

RHEUMATOID ARTHRITIS

This illness most often attacks those in their thirties or forties. It is more common in women than men. Of all the rheumatic diseases this is one of the most serious and crippling. There is some evidence that it is associated with a bacterial infection.

Onset of the disease is generally accompanied by pain and swellings in the fingers and this may eventually spread throughout the joints of the body. Rheumatoid arthritis attacks may be accompanied by fever, and if the attack is serious the fever can be equally severe.

The characteristic appearance of the hands is a pulling of the fingers towards the small finger and an enlargement of the joints with wasting of the muscles in between.

Rest, gentle exercise and heat are all of benefit in a general regimen of treatment which should include use of some of the recommended herbs.

OSTEOARTHRITIS

Present in a high proportion of older people, this joint disorder is often brought about by pre-existing injury — although it is sometimes thought to be hereditary. Osteoarthritis is a degenerative condition, but is characterised by periods of remission which can often cause confusion when they occur during times of medical treatment.

The action of the condition is to gradually destroy the central part of the cartilage of the affected joint — and at the same time the outer part grows over the joint. Eventually, bony spurs, known as osteophytes, occur.

Osteoarthritis most commonly affects the joints of the shoulder, hip and knee and also the end joints of the fingers.

Rest, gentle exercise and heat are of benefit together with treatment by use of the appropriate herbs. When excess weight is a problem this should be eliminated by dieting to take pressure off the affected joints. Diet can also play an important part in treatment.

Chapter 2

Some Commonly Used Drugs

This chapter outlines some of the drugs prescribed by doctors for the treatment of rheumatism, arthritis and other musculo-skeletal diseases, together with some of the side effects and adverse reactions associated with them. Some of the drugs listed in the first edition of this book have been withdrawn, or reformulated, or have been replaced by more modern preparations.

The information has not been given to alarm anyone who may be taking any of these drugs, but to make them aware of their possible effects. However, it should be emphasised that people react differently to drugs and that not everyone will, necessarily, suffer side effects.

I believe that many doctors fail to explain fully to their patients the side effects that can be expected from a particular drug, or course of treatment, and that this may cause great distress. This is often due to a failure to communicate since pharmaceutical companies usually advise doctors of the side effects reported during the clinical trials of their medicines.

While there are a number of drugs used for rheumatic and arthritic diseases which are not listed here, and which are deemed to have fewer side effects, it should be remembered that all chemical-based drugs are expected to produce side effects.

There is often more than one proprietary brand of a drug, particularly where the patent for the original drug has expired. Brand names are given in brackets.

BENORYLATE
(Benoral)

Indications: Rheumatoid arthritis, osteoarthritis and other painful musculoskeletal conditions.

Possible side effects: Gastrointestinal upset, asthma.

DIFLUNISAL
(Dolobid)

Indications: Rheumatoid arthritis and osteoarthritis.

Possible side effects: Gastric disturbance, stomach pain, indigestion, tinnitus, diarrhoea.

FENOPROFEN
(Fenopron)

Indications: Rheumatoid arthritis, osteoarthritis, ankylosing spondylitis.

Possible side effects: Gastric disturbances, allergies, liver and kidney disorders, asthma.

FLURBIPROFEN
(Froben)

Indications: Rheumatoid arthritis, osteoarthritis, ankylosing spondylitis.

Possible side effects: Gastric upset, rashes, oedema, asthma.

IBUPROFEN
(Brufen)

Indications: Adult and juvenile rheumatoid arthritis, osteoarthritis, ankylosing spondylitis, soft tissue injuries.

Possible side effects: Gastric bleeding, indigestion, asthma, rash.

INDOMETHACIN
(Indocid)

Indications: Acute gout, rheumatoid arthritis, osteoarthritis, ankylosing spondylitis, acute joint disorders.

Possible side effects: Headaches, gastric bleeding, dizziness, rashes, eye disturbances, some blood disorders. May also interact with other drugs.

KETOPROFEN
(Orudis)

Indications: Rheumatoid arthritis, osteoarthrosis, ankylosing spondylitis, acute joint disease, acute gout.

Possible side effects: Gastric upsets, rashes. May interact with other drugs.

MEFENAMIC ACID
(Ponstan Forte)

Indications: Painful rheumatoid arthritis and Still's disease, and osteoarthrosis.

| **Possible side effects:** | Diarrhoea, skin rash. May also affect kidneys and blood. |

NAPROXEN
(Naprosyn)

| **Indications:** | Acute gout, ankylosing spondylitis, rheumatoid arthritis, osteoarthritis. |
| **Possible side effects:** | Gastric disturbances, rashes, headaches, tinnitus, vertigo, blood disorders. |

PREDNISONE
(Decortisyl)

| **Indications:** | Rheumatic conditions. |
| **Possible side effects:** | Peptic ulceration, mood changes, osteoporosis. |

PREDNISOLONE
(Deltacortril)
(Prednesol)

| **Indications:** | Rheumatic conditions. |
| **Possible side effects:** | Similar to prednisone. |

SODIUM AUROTHIOMALATE
(Myocrisin)

| **Indications:** | Rheumatoid arthritis. |
| **Possible side effects:** | This drug (a gold salt) is given by injection. The treatment can induce diarrhoea, itching, bruising, rashes, heavy menstrual periods, and a metallic taste. It may also affect the blood and urine. |

SULINDAC
(Clinoril)

Indications: Acute gout and joint conditions, ankylosing spondylitis, rheumatoid arthritis, osteoarthrosis.

Possible side effects: Stomach pain, indigestion, bitter taste in mouth, tinnitus, dizziness, sore tongue, asthma, visual disturbance, blood disorders.

TRIAMCINOLONE
(Adcortyl)
(Ledercort)

Indications: Painful, stiff and swollen joints associated with rheumatoid arthritis and osteoarthritis.

Possible side effects: Dizziness, muscle weakness, sleepiness, flushing.

Chapter 3

Some Problems which Trouble Sufferers

One of the worst features of rheumatism and arthritis, apart from the pain and stiffness involved, is their tendency to incapacitate by causing malformation of the hands and limbs. This can lead to people having to give up their jobs and to discontinuing favourite hobbies such as sewing and knitting.

There can be no doubt that one of the greatest advances in recent years has been the technique of joint replacement, which has given mobility back to many sufferers who had become confined to wheelchairs, or dependent on walking sticks. However, merely to replace an affected part does not halt the disease, and many people have found changes even of the artificial joints necessary. Therefore, it can be seen that internal control of the factors causing the progression of the illness become all-important.

While causes leading to the start of these illnesses can often be pin-pointed, it is still not generally understood why some people are more prone than others — or why a more marked and rapid deterioration occurs in some cases.

Interestingly, rheumatoid arthritis has for many years been linked by some researchers with an excess of static electricity in the body, and when that is relieved there is often a lessening of the pain and discomfort. For this reason, many sufferers can be seen wearing a small copper wrist-bangle, which has the effect of 'earthing' the body. Similarly for many years, my father recommended to patients that they walk barefoot on the lawn several times daily, and in many cases great relief was reported to him.

Medical practitioners may be sceptical of such methods, but in the absence of a safe 'modern' cure or treatment, such an attitude is really not called for. All treatments which can claim a success rate are deserving of study — and a copper bracelet has certainly never killed anyone — which is more than can be said for some recently prescribed chemical drugs.

Herbal medicine has always concerned itself with a balanced treatment of an individual's ills, and it is for this reason that other aspects of the problem are looked at when a herbal practitioner makes recommendations.

With rheumatism and arthritis I have always found depression and mental tension to be serious side effects, and effective treatment for them will often change patients' outlooks and allow them to face the future with more confidence. There are many safe herbal treatments available for tension, some of them shown in the herb section of this book and others covered in a companion volume *Stress and Tension*.

Another noticeable side effect is poor circulation. Here again, herbal treatment can be very effective and I would strongly recommend Vitamin E and any herbal tablets containing Rutin.

Chapter 4

The Importance of Diet

During consultations, I am often asked to give detailed diets. My answer to this is normally to suggest items best avoided for a particular illness, but to leave the actual details of the food to the patient's own good sense.

Putting it quite simply, if you suffer from a stomach ulcer and fried foods aggravate it, you should avoid them in the future. Similarly with most other illnesses, if certain food or drinks inflame and intensify the condition, then this is normally sufficient to act as a deterrent.

With rheumatism and arthritis, I have found from experience that certain foods and drinks should not be taken regularly in the diet, since they can have an adverse effect. Those with a high acid content are best avoided. By this I mean citrus fruits and drinks (fresh orange, lemon, lime, grapefruit, rhubarb). Also, many greens, such as spring greens, Brussels sprouts and sometimes lettuce can have an adverse effect.

The main thing to avoid is a high concentration and, therefore, occasional use will probably be of no harm. Generally, a high protein diet should be avoided, particularly too much meat. Plenty of vegetables should be eaten. Following these simple diet suggestions can greatly help both conditions — and, of course, an avoidance of alcohol is also strongly recommended. Drink plenty of milk and eat small amounts regularly and often, avoiding very large meals.

Chapter 5

Herbal Treatments and Medication

The formulae in this chapter are all suitable to make at home following the given instructions and using quantities shown as percentages of the overall herb weight.

Ingredients should be available from medical herbalists, herbal retailers and many health food shops — if any difficulty is experienced consult the list of addresses at the back of the book.

INFORMATION ON THE PREPARATION OF HERBS

DECOCTIONS
The herbs are cut, ground up or bruised and covered with cold fresh water. This mixture is then boiled for up to half an hour, allowed to cool and then strained through a fine mesh. Allow 28 grams of the herbs to 568 ml of water (1 oz to 1 pint). This method is normally used when the herb is unsuitable to make as an infusion. The usual dose is approximately one small wineglassful three times daily.

INFUSIONS
Teas or tisanes are made by the process of infusion. Prepare the herbs to be used and quickly pour boiling water on them. Allow the mixture to stand for about

half an hour, stirring frequently, and when ready, strain off the liquid. Allow 28 grams to 568 ml of water (1 oz to 1 pint). The usual dose is approximately one small teacup or wineglassful three times daily, usually one after each main meal.

SOLID EXTRACTS
Start with a strong infusion of the herbs required and evaporate over low heat until a heavy consistency is obtained.

TINCTURES
This process is used for herbs and drugs which become useless when heated, or for those herbs which are not amenable to treatment by water. Tinctures are made commercially with pure alcohol. Use 28 to 56 grams to 568 ml (1 or 2 oz to 1 pint). The dose varies according to the strength of the main ingredient. For home use tinctures can be made with brandy, but this is rather an expensive process.

SOME SIMPLE FORMULAE TO MAKE AT HOME

A GOOD GENERAL HERB MIXTURE FOR RHEUMATISM

Oats (Avena)	1 part
Dandelion Root	1 part
Paraguay Tea (Maté)	2 parts
Heather Flowers	1 part

Make up as an infusion.

A HERB MIXTURE FOR FIBROSITIS AND LUMBAGO

Sweet Chestnut	1 part
Devil's Claw	1 part

Make up as an infusion.

A HERB MIXTURE FOR MYALGIA

Buckbean	1 part
Meadowsweet	1 part
Black Cohosh	1 part

Make up as an infusion.

A HERB MIXTURE FOR MUSCULAR RHEUMATISM

Wild Yam Root	1 part
Devil's Claw	1 part
Buckbean	1 part
Black Cohosh	1 part

Make up as an infusion.

A HERB MIXTURE FOR RHEUMATOID ARTHRITIS

Celery Seed	2 parts
Meadowsweet	1 part
White Willow Bark	1 part
Wild Yam Root	1 part

Make up as an infusion.

AN ALTERNATIVE HERB MIXTURE FOR RHEUMATOID ARTHRITIS

Agrimony	1 part
Sarsaparilla	1 part
White Poplar	1 part
Meadowsweet	1 part

Make up as an infusion.

A HERB MIXTURE FOR GOUT

Gravel Root	1 part
Burdock	1 part
Dandelion Root	1 part
Meadowsweet	1 part

Make up as a decoction.

A HERB MIXTURE FOR SCIATICA

Burdock Root	1 part
Buckbean	1 part
Meadowsweet	1 part
St John's Wort	1 part

Make up as an infusion.

A GENERAL HERB POULTICE FOR EXTERNAL
RHEUMATIC AND JOINT INFLAMMATION —
ALSO HELPFUL FOR GOUT

Fenugreek Seeds	1 part
Savory, Summer	2 parts
Capsicum	1 part
Marshmallow	2 parts
Mustard Seeds	1 part

Mix with hot water to make a comfortable warm poultice and loosely bind over affected area.

Chapter 6

Some Recommended Herbs

This section lists herbs which have been used by medical herbalists in the treatment of arthritis and rheumatism, together with other herbs which have a general toning effect on the whole body.

Caution: Due to the need for accurate dosage, many of these herbs may be available only on prescription from a medical herbalist and should not be picked from the wild. Neither should garden varieties be used. They are included for information only.

A list of suppliers is given at the end of the section.

Acacia Gum
ACACIA SENEGAL

Also known as	Gum Arabic.
Where found	North Africa.
Appearance	Round tears obtained from spring shrub. Cuts are made in the bark and the gum exudes and coagulates.
Part used	Coagulated gum.
Therapeutic uses	An excellent demulcent, often used to relieve catarrh and chest complaints.
Prepared as	Mucilage by combining with hot water.

Adder's Tongue (American)
ERYTHRONIUM AMERICANUM

Also known as	Snake's Tongue.
Where found	North America.
Appearance	Small bulbous plant with only two leaves; bright yellow lily-like flowers.
Part used	Leaves.
Therapeutic uses	Generally as a poultice for ulcers and skin troubles.
Prepared as	Poultice.

Agar-Agar
GELIDIUM AMANSII

Also known as	Japanese Isinglass.
Where found	Japan.
Appearance	Prepared from a compound of several different seaweeds into thin strips of about 30 cm (12 ins) long from dried jelly.
Part used	Translucent strips.
Therapeutic uses	Excellent for relief of stubborn constipation.
Prepared as	Powder.

Agrimony
AGRIMONIA EUPATORIA

Also known as	Church Steeples

Where found	Throughout Northern Europe.
Appearance	A strong growing herb with green-grey leaves covered with soft hairs. Flowers are small and yellow on long slender spikes.
Part used	Herb.
Therapeutic uses	Dried leaves when infused make a good general tonic for the whole system. At one time it was so revered that it was used as a remedy for practically every ill. It is still used as a remedy for rheumatoid arthritis. The infusion taken internally, or applied externally in the form of a compress, improves skin function, helping to clear pustular eruptions, pimples and blotches. The dried leaves infused are useful for treating diarrhoea and general intestinal debility, and to help prevent tissue wasting due to malabsorption.
Prepared as	Infusion, tincture.

Alder, English
ALNUS GLUTINOSA

Where found	England, Europe and North Africa.
Appearance	A small tree of distinctive appearance.
Parts used	Bark and leaves.

Therapeutic uses   The bark is used as a cathartic
                       and the leaves to treat
                       inflammatory conditions.

Prepared as   Poultice.

Amaranth
AMARANTHUS HYPOCHONDRIACUS

Also known as   Love Lies Bleeding.
Where found   UK and Europe.
Appearance   A common garden plant with
                       crimson flowers similar to a
                       coxscomb.
Part used   Herb.
Therapeutic uses   Treatment of diarrhoea and
                       menorrhagia. As an astringent.
                       Helpful in all cases of looseness of
                       the bowel.
Prepared as   Decoction.

Angelica
ANGELICA ARCHANGELICA

Where found   Europe, Asia.
Appearance   Plant growing from one and a half
                       to two metres high.
Parts used   Root, seeds and herb.

Therapeutic uses	A stimulant and diaphoretic used for rheumatic diseases, catarrh and asthma. It can be seen from its name that this herb has strong religious connections. It is said that the properties of the plant were revealed by an angel in a dream, and it was reputed to be able to cure the plague. An infusion to which honey and lemon is added is taken in small doses as a treatment for feverish conditions.
Prepared as	Infusion or decoction.

Aniseed
PIMPINELLA ANISUM

Where found	Europe and North Africa.
Appearance	An umbelliferous plant with serrated leaves. Small brownish-grey seeds.
Part used	Fruit.
Therapeutic uses	A pectoral. Used for cough medicines and elixirs.
Prepared as	Powder or decoction.

Avens
GEUM URBANUM

Also known as	Colewort.
Where found	Throughout Europe.

Appearance	Low-growing herb with yellow flowers.
Parts used	Herb and root.
Therapeutic uses	The plant is astringent, antiseptic, and aromatic, and has a number of uses, including its ability to stop cuts and wounds from bleeding. It is a good stomach and bowel tonic, particularly where there is much distension and flatulence, or where there is ulceration. It has also been used for treating leucorrhoea in women. As a digestive tonic it can be combined with raspberry and agrimony, or with angelica.
Prepared as	Decoction.

Balm of Gilead
POPULUS CANDICANS

Also known as	Several other plants are known as Balm of Gilead.
Where found	United States and Arabia.
Appearance	Strong gnarled shrub with feathery foliage.
Part used	Buds.
Therapeutic uses	Highly regarded as a tonic and diuretic. Excellent for chest troubles and rheumatic ailments.

| **Prepared as** | Decoction or tincture. |

Balmony
CHELONE GLABRA

Also known as	Turtle Head, Snake Herb.
Where found	United States and Canada.
Appearance	Low sturdy bush with oval dark leaves and white or pink flowers.
Part used	Leaves.
Therapeutic uses	Regarded as one of the best remedies for liver diseases. It is also antibilious, anthelmintic and a tonic.
Prepared as	Infusion.

Bayberry
MYRICA CERIFERA

Also known as	Waxberry, Candleberry.
Where found	Europe and North America.
Appearance	A medium-growing shrub with a profusion of large white berries.
Part used	Bark.
Therapeutic uses	A strong stimulant. A warming and effective deobstruent and cleanser. Small doses only. Also as a poultice for ulcers.
Prepared as	Infusion and poultice.

Bearsfoot, American
POLYMNIA UVEDALIA

Also known as	Yellow Leaf Cup.
Where found	North America.
Appearance	A tall branching plant found in rich loamy soil.
Part used	Root.
Therapeutic uses	Regarded as a valuable aid for quick pain relief, as a gentle laxative for the aged and as a stimulant.
Prepared as	Decoction.

Birch, European
BETULA ALBA

Where found	Europe.
Appearance	A strikingly handsome tree common on gravel soils. Distinctive black and white bark.
Parts used	Bark and leaves.
Therapeutic uses	Birch tar oil makes a soothing ointment for skin disorders. The bark, as an infusion, is good for kidney stones.
Prepared as	Ointment.

Bistort
POLYGONUM BISTORTA

Also known as	Adderwort.

Where found	Europe and northern Britain.
Appearance	Low-growing herb chiefly found in ditches and damp places.
Part used	Root.
Therapeutic uses	Regarded as effective in incontinence and as a gargle for sore throats.
Prepared as	Decoction.

Black Root
LEPTANDRA VIRGINICA

Also known as	Culver's Root.
Where found	United States.
Appearance	A low-growing herb.
Part used	Rhizome.
Therapeutic uses	A blood purifying mixture. Also as a cathartic, diaphoretic and a liver stimulant.
Prepared as	Decoction.

Bladderwrack
FUCUS VESICULOSUS

Also known as	Seawrack and Kelpware.
Where found	Around coasts of Britain.
Appearance	A large trailing dark green seaweed.
Part used	Dried plant.
Therapeutic uses	Acts on thyroid. Tones up the system and clears the kidneys.

Prepared as	Decoction.

Blue Flag
IRIS VERSICOLOR

Also known as	Flag Lily, Water Flag.
Where found	Extensively planted in gardens throughout Britain.
Appearance	A beautiful plant with arching strap-like leaves and blue, white, yellow or multi-colour flowers.
Part used	Rhizome.
Therapeutic uses	Principally as a blood purifier, also an alterative, diuretic and cathartic.
Prepared as	Decoction or powder. Small doses only.

Borage
BORAGO OFFICINALIS

Also known as	Burrage.
Where found	Throughout Europe.
Appearance	Bold, erect herb of strong growth. Small blue flowers.
Part used	Leaves.
Therapeutic uses	As a diuretic and demulcent and a flavouring agent.
Prepared as	Infusion and poultice.

Boxwood, American
CORNUS FLORIDA

Also known as	Dogwood, Cornel.
Where found	United States.
Appearance	Small tree with rough bark and a profusion of pink spring flowers.
Parts used	Root and bark.
Therapeutic uses	As a tonic and stimulant, also as a remedy for migraine and headaches.
Prepared as	Decoction or powder.

Broom
CYTISUS SCOPARIUS

Also known as	Irish Broom.
Where found	Throughout Europe.
Appearance	A small graceful arching shrub with profuse floral display.
Part used	Top of each sprig.
Therapeutic uses	As a diuretic and cathartic. Also for relief of liver troubles and fluid retention. May affect blood pressure. Only use under the supervision of a qualified practitioner.
Prepared as	Infusion.

Buchu

BAROSMA BETULINA

Also known as	Bucco.
Where found	Western coast of South Africa.
Appearance	Small procumbent herb growing in dry places.
Part used	Leaves.
Therapeutic uses	Urinary and bladder troubles. Also a diaphoretic and stimulant. Buchu has an antiseptic action on the whole of the urinary tract and is employed in mixtures for the treatment of inflammatory bladder conditions, such as cystitis. It is often combined with other more soothing remedies, such as Marshmallow and Corn Silk, and with small amounts of more stimulating remedies, such as Couch Grass and Juniper.
Prepared as	Infusion or decoction.

Buckbean

MENYANTHES TRIFOLIATA

Also known as	Bogbean, Marsh Trefoil.
Where found	UK and Europe.
Appearance	Aquatic plant.
Part used	Herb.
Therapeutic uses	Muscular rheumatism and rheumatoid arthritis.
Prepared as	Decoction.

Bugle
AJUGA REPTANS

Also known as	Sicklewort.
Where found	European woodlands.
Appearance	Diminutive herb with distinctive square stems and blue flowers.
Part used	Herb.
Therapeutic use	An astringent.
Prepared as	Infusion.

Bugloss
ECHIUM VULGARE

Also known as	Viper's Bugloss.
Where found	Europe.
Appearance	A sturdy herb with blue flowers.
Part used	Herb.
Therapeutic uses	An expectorant and demulcent. Excellent for gentle bowel action. Also to clear phlegm from bronchial tubes.
Prepared as	Infusion.

Burdock
ARCTIUM LAPPA

Also known as	Lappa.
Where found	UK and Europe.

Appearance	Herb growing to as high as one and a half metres, with large rhubarb-shaped leaves.
Part used	Herb, root and seeds.
Therapeutic uses	Rheumatism, gout, skin eruptions. Also a diuretic.
Prepared as	Decoction.

Cajaput
MELALEUCA LEUCADENDRON

Also known as	White Tea Tree.
Where found	East Indies.
Appearance	A big bold tree.
Part used	Oil.
Therapeutic uses	For rheumatism and bruises. Also rubbed onto the gums for toothache.
Prepared as	Oil, as a rub for external use.

Canella
CANELLA ALBA

Also known as	Wild Cinnamon.
Where found	West Indies.
Appearance	Slender branching tree with light grey bark.
Part used	Bark.

Therapeutic uses	Stimulant tonic for the aged. Promotes digestion and elimination and prevents flatulence.
Prepared as	Decoction.

Capsicum
CAPSICUM MINIMUM

Also known as	Cayenne, Chillies.
Where found	Tropical countries including Africa and South America.
Appearance	Small shrub with red fruits.
Part used	Fruit.
Therapeutic uses	An intensely stimulating agent which is used in very small doses only. It is used in external lotions, plasters and ointments for lumbago or sciatica, and taken internally in small doses, usually in mixtures made up for arthritis and rheumatism, to increase blood circulation through the joints. It is warming to the whole system and one or two doses of the powder can relieve a cold. It is also included in digestive remedies in small amounts when a carminative is indicated.
Prepared as	Powder, pills, tincture.

Catnip
NEPETA CATARIA

Also known as	Catmint.
Where found	Britain.
Appearance	A procumbent grey plant.
Part used	Herb.
Therapeutic uses	Carminative and diaphoretic and has tonic properties. Also used for the relief of piles. It combines well with other digestive remedies such as agrimony, chamomile and dandelion when made up into an infusion. For piles, the leaves are incorporated into an ointment, or made into an infused oil and a little inserted into the rectum. The infusion is also used to relieve headache. In large doses Catnip tends to be emetic and may induce vomiting.
Prepared as	Infusion.

Cayenne, Hungarian
CAPSICUM TETRAGONUM

Also known as	Paprika.
Where found	Hungary, also cultivated elsewhere.
Appearance	A strong-growing herb with large green fruits.

Part used	Fruit.
Therapeutic uses	Rich source of vitamin C.
Prepared as	Powder. Small doses.

Celery
APIUM GRAVEOLENS

Where found	Europe.
Appearance	This is the familiar vegetable.
Parts used	Stem and seeds.
Therapeutic uses	A tonic diuretic and carminative and an aid for rheumatoid troubles. Also regarded as an effective aphrodisiac.
Prepared as	Decoction or powder from the seeds.

Chamomile, Belgian
ANTHEMIS NOBILIS

Where found	Belgium and France. Widely cultivated.
Appearance	Herb with double flowers.
Part used	Flowers.
Therapeutic uses	Widely used for women suffering from nervous upsets and as a tonic, stomachic and antispasmodic.
Prepared as	Infusion.

Chamomile, German
MATRICARIA CHAMOMILLA

Where found	Europe.
Appearance	Herb with small cushion-like flowers in profusion.
Part used	Flowers.
Therapeutic uses	Excellent nerve sedative, carminative and tonic.
Prepared as	Infusion.

Chickweed
STELLARIA MEDIA

Also known as	Starweed.
Where found	Britain.
Appearance	Small prolific weed.
Part used	Herb.
Therapeutic uses	A demulcent and to allay feverish conditions.
Prepared as	Decoction.

Cinnamon
CINNAMOMUM ZEYLANICUM

Where found	A native plant of Ceylon.
Appearance	A tree growing up to 30ft high in sandy soils.
Part used	Bark.
Therapeutic uses	Very effective for treating vomiting and nausea, and will relieve flatulence and diarrhoea.
Prepared as	Medicinal water, tincture, powder.

Cohosh, Black
CIMICIFUGA RACEMOSA

Also known as	Squaw Root
Where found	United States and Canada.
Appearance	A tall herbaceous plant with white feathery flowers.
Part used	Rhizome.
Therapeutic uses	A herb used for rheumatic conditions. It is antispasmodic, sedative, astringent, a blood purifier and nervine. Used in small doses for loose bowel and diarrhoea. Large doses may cause nausea and vomiting. It is antiflatulent. The Red Indians of North America used it to treat various menstrual complaints, and in recent times, it has been found to contain active principles resembling oestrogen.
Prepared as	Decoction. Avoid in pregnancy. Best taken under supervision of a herbalist.

Cohosh, Blue
CAULOPHYLLUM THALICTROIDES

Also known as	Blueberry Root.
Where found	United States and Canada.

Appearance	A gnarled, crowded shrub.
Part used	Rhizome.
Therapeutic uses	As a diuretic and emmenagogue and also as a vermifuge to expel worms. Aids rheumatic sufferers and menstrual problems.
Prepared as	Decoction. Avoid in pregnancy. Use small doses only.

Comfrey
SYMPHYTUM OFFICINALE

Also known as	Knitbone and Slippery Root.
Where found	Throughout the UK and Europe.
Appearance	Fleshy-leaved plant which can grow to about one metre.
Parts used	Leaves and root.
Therapeutic uses	Helpful for treatment of leg ulcers. For rheumatic pains and for arthritis, and a poultice for treatment of bruises and sprains.
Prepared as	Ointment, poultice and infused oil for external use.

Cornsilk
ZEA MAYS

Where found	South Africa and America.
Appearance	Maize.
Part used	Part of flower.

Therapeutic uses	Principally as a diuretic but also for pulmonary troubles. It is known among herbalists as the 'brick dust remover' because it is an excellent remedy for those inclined to form gravel in the urine. The tincture is given in combination with tincture of couch grass.
Prepared as	Decoction.

Cotton Root
GOSSYPIUM HERBACEUM

Where found	Mediterranean islands and the United States.
Appearance	Twist of bark.
Part used	Bark of root.
Therapeutic uses	Emmenagogue.
Prepared as	Infusion. Avoid in pregnancy.

Couchgrass
AGROPYRON REPENS

Also known as	Twitchgrass.
Where found	In most parts of the world.

Appearance	A strong grass with white fleshy roots.
Part used	Rhizome.
Therapeutic uses	For treatment of cystitis, nephritis and bladder troubles. Also for rheumatoid ills and as a diuretic and aperient.
Prepared as	Infusion.

Cramp Bark
VIBURNUM OPULUS

Also known as	Snow-ball Tree, Guelder Rose.
Where found	Europe and America.
Appearance	Strong-growing bush with white ball-shaped flowers.
Part used	Bark.
Therapeutic uses	As a nervine for treatment of cramping pains, spasms and convulsions. Antispasmodic.
Prepared as	Decoction.

Cranesbill, American
GERANIUM MACULATUM

Also known as	Wild Geranium, Storksbill.
Where found	United States.
Appearance	Shrubby small herb with blue flowers.

50

Parts used	Herb and root.
Therapeutic uses	Has quick styptic properties and is a tonic and astringent. Treatment for piles and ulcers.
Prepared as	Decoction.

Damiana
TURNERA DIFFUSA

Where found	Southern United States and Mexico.
Appearance	Medium-sized shrub.
Parts used	Leaves and stem.
Therapeutic uses	Famous for its aphrodisiac qualities. As a tonic for the aged and those suffering from exhaustion and debility.
Prepared as	Infusion.

Dandelion
TARAXACUM OFFICINALE

Where found	Most temperate climates.
Appearance	Common herb with long root, toothed leaves and bright yellow flowers.
Parts used	Leaves and root.
Therapeutic uses	As a tonic and diuretic and for liver and kidney ills. Roots frequently used for coffee as it contains no caffeine.
Prepared as	Infusion or decoction.

Devil's Claw
HARPAGOPHYTUM PROCUMBENS

Where found	Southern part of Africa.
Appearance	Low-growing plant.
Part used	Root.
Therapeutic uses	Of great value for the treatment of inflammatory and rheumatic conditions. Also has sedative and diuretic properties.
Prepared as	Decoction.

Dog Rose
ROSA CANINA

Also known as	Wild Briar.
Where found	Europe and the Middle East.
Appearance	The wild rambling rose.
Part used	Fruit.
Therapeutic uses	The fruit yields ascorbic acid (vitamin C) of great value when given to young children.
Prepared as	Rose hip syrup.

Echinacea
ECHINACEA ANGUSTIFOLIA

Also known as	Coneflower.
Where found	United States.

Appearance	Herb of medium height.
Part used	Rhizome.
Therapeutic uses	As an antiseptic and alterative and to help purify the blood. Useful agent in infections.
Prepared as	Decoction.

Elder
SAMBUCUS NIGRA

Also known as	Black Elder.
Where found	Europe.
Appearance	A tall straggling shrub with profuse crops of black berries.
Parts used	Flowers, berries and bark.
Therapeutic uses	For colds and influenza. As an alterative and diuretic. It is a safe soporific and induces healthy sleep.
Prepared as	Infusion.

Evening Primrose
OENOTHERA BIENNIS

Also known as	Tree Primrose.
Where found	European gardens.
Appearance	A small herb with a delightful display of yellow flowers.
Parts used	Leaves, bark and oil.
Therapeutic uses	As a sedative and astringent. For the relief of female menstrual disorders. The oil gives relief in arthritic conditions.

Prepared as   Decoction. The oil is available in capsules.

Fenugreek
TRIGONELLA FOENUM-GRAECUM

Where found	Mediterranean area, North Africa and India.
Appearance	Slender stemmed plant.
Part used	Herb.
Therapeutic uses	As an emollient, a laxative and expectorant. Can be applied externally to assist gout.
Prepared as	Decoction and poultice.

Feverfew
CHRYSANTHEMUM PARTHENIUM

Also known as	Featherfew.
Where found	Throughout Europe.
Appearance	A small grey herb with hairy stems.
Part used	Herb.
Therapeutic uses	As an aperient, also used by women to bring on the menses. Now recognised as an aid to migraine.
Prepared as	Infusion, tablets. Contraindicated in pregnancy.

Figwort
SCROPHULARIA NODOSA

Also known as	Throatwort.
Where found	Throughout Europe.
Appearance	Medium-sized tree of rampant growth.
Part used	Herb.
Therapeutic uses	Aperient, also an emollient and demulcent and as a poultice for ulcers.
Prepared as	Infusion and poultice.

Fringetree
CHIONANTHUS VIRGINICA

Where found	Southern United States.
Appearance	A small tree with inconspicuous white flowers. It has a very bitter taste.
Part used	The bark of the root.
Therapeutic uses	Tonic, alterative and diuretic. Also for the treatment of liver disorders, gallstones and jaundice.
Prepared as	Decoction. Small doses only.

Garlic
ALLIUM SATIVUM

Where found	Universally cultivated.
Appearance	Similar to a shallot.

Part used	Bulb.
Therapeutic uses	For treatment of dyspepsia and flatulence, also as a stimulant; garlic is a powerful antiseptic and anti-infective agent and is taken internally as a preventive treatment against colds and flu and to treat a wide range of infections. It has also been found to lower blood cholesterol levels and thus helps protect against heart disease. Odour-free and odour-controlled garlic preparations are now available from health food stores.
Prepared as	Juice and tincture.

Gentian
GENTIANA LUTEA

Where found	Alpine meadows.
Appearance	A plant with oblong, pale green leaves and large, yellow scented flowers.
Part used	Root.
Therapeutic use	Tonic. It is very bitter and only small doses are required.
Prepared as	Decoction or powder.

Ginger
ZINGIBER OFFICINALE

Where found	West Indies and China.
Appearance	About one metre high with glossy aromatic leaves.
Part used	Rhizome.
Therapeutic uses	Has stimulative and carminative properties and can be used as an expectorant and digestive aid.
Prepared as	Powder or decoction. Only small doses are used.

Ginseng
PANAX QUINQUEFOLIUM

Also known as	Chinese Panacea, Panax.
Where found	China and Mongolia.
Appearance	Erect-growing herb with vivid fleshy leaves.
Part used	Root.
Therapeutic uses	Tonic, aids fertility. Also aids digestive problems.
Prepared as	Powder or decoction.

Golden Seal
HYDRASTIS CANADENSIS

Also known as	Yellow Root.

Where found	Cultivated in North America.
Appearance	Tall-growing herb with disagreeable odour.
Part used	Rhizome.
Therapeutic uses	For gastric disorders and as a soothing laxative and tonic.
Prepared as	Decoction or powder. Small doses only. Contraindicated in pregnancy.

Goutwort
AEGOPODIUM PODAGRARIA

Also known as	Goutweed.
Where found	Throughout Europe.
Appearance	A small spreading herb.
Part used	Herb.
Therapeutic uses	For the relief of sciatica and gout; of value when used as a poultice.
Prepared as	Poultice.

Gravel Root
EUPATORIUM PURPUREUM

Also known as	Gravel Weed.
Where found	North America.
Appearance	Herb growing to about a metre high.
Part used	Rhizome.
Therapeutic uses	Diuretic and anti-rheumatic. Helpful in gout, rheumatism, kidney stones and cystitis.

Prepared as   Decoction.

Guaiacum
GUAIACUM OFFICINALE

Also known as	Lignum Vitae.
Where found	West Indies and South America.
Appearance	A strong tree producing the strongest wood in the world.
Parts used	Wood and resin.
Therapeutic uses	For the relief of rheumatism, and as a diaphoretic and alterative.
Prepared as	Decoction.

Guarana
PAULLINIA CUPANA

Also known as	Brazilian Cocoa.
Where found	Brazil.
Appearance	A tall arching shrub.
Part used	Seeds.
Therapeutic uses	As a stimulant and for relief of headaches and migraine. Also used by women to bring on menses and can be effective in treatment of arthritis.
Prepared as	Decoction or powder.

Hawthorn
CRATAEGUS OXYCANTHA

Also known as	May Tree.
Where found	Throughout Britain.
Appearance	A common small tree.
Part used	Fruit.
Therapeutic use	As an aid for heart conditions.
Prepared as	Decoction. Use under the supervision of a practitioner.

Heather Flowers
CALLUNA VULGARIS

Also known as	Ling Flowers.
Where found	UK and Europe.
Appearance	Evergreen shrub.
Part used	Flowers.
Therapeutic uses	Has anti-rheumatic properties and is also a diuretic. Has proved useful in cases of cystitis, gout and rheumatic pains.
Prepared as	Infusion.

Hops
HUMULUS LUPULUS

Where found	Europe, and cultivated in most parts of the world.
Appearance	A climbing vine.

Part used	Strobiles.
Therapeutic uses	As an anodyne for the relief of pain. Also as a tonic and an aid for stomach disorders and to promote sleep.
Prepared as	Infusion. Small doses only.

Horseradish
COCHLEARIA ARMORACIA

Where found	Europe.
Appearance	A herb growing to one metre with a pungent odour.
Part used	Root.
Therapeutic uses	Relieves flatulence and indigestion. Promotes perspiration and is a diuretic.
Prepared as	Infusion.

Horsetail
EQUISETUM ARVENSE

Also known as	Scouring Rushes.
Where found	Britain.
Appearance	A tall bold herb with cane-like appearance.
Part used	Herb.
Therapeutic uses	A powerful astringent and also a diuretic. Excellent for kidney troubles.
Prepared as	Decoction.

Houndstongue
CYNOGLOSSUM OFFICINALE

Where found	Britain.
Appearance	A medium-sized herb with long, strap-like leaves.
Part used	Herb.
Therapeutic uses	An anodyne for relief of pain. Also as a demulcent for soothing coughs and colds. Can also be used to reduce piles.
Prepared as	Infusion.

Houseleek
SEMPERVIVUM TECTORUM

Where found	Throughout Britain.
Appearance	Small procumbent plant.
Part used	Leaves.
Therapeutic uses	As an astringent and poultice. Commonly used to soften corns and hard skin.
Prepared as	Poultice.

Hyssop
HYSSSOPUS OFFICINALIS

Where found	U.K.
Appearance	Small common field herb.
Part used	Leaves.

| **Therapeutic uses** | Stimulant and carminative for bronchial and nasal catarrah. Also for anxiety states and tension. |
| **Prepared as** | Infusion. |

Iceland Moss
CETRARIA ISLANDICA

Where found	Throughout the northern hemisphere.
Appearance	This is not a moss but a procumbent grey lichen.
Part used	Plant.
Therapeutic uses	For catarrh and bronchitis. It is a nutritive and helpful for digestive complaints.
Prepared as	Decoction.

Irish Moss
CHONDRUS CRISPUS

Also known as	Carragheen Moss
Where found	European and North American coasts.
Appearance	Small, procumbent seaweed with fan-shaped fronds.
Part used	Whole plant.
Therapeutic uses	Mainly in cough medicines for its demulcent properties. It is nutritious and can be used as a food. Externally as a lotion for dermatitis and roughened hands.
Prepared as	Decoction.

Jambul

EUGENIA JAMBOLANA

Also known as	Java Plum.
Where found	East India.
Appearance	A large spreading tree.
Part used	Seeds.
Therapeutic uses	Helpful to diabetics. Reduces sugar content of urine.
Prepared as	Decoction.

Juniper

JUNIPERUS COMMUNIS

Where found	Europe and Asia.
Appearance	A bush or tree up to 3 metres in height producing dark purple berries.
Part used	Berry.
Therapeutic uses	Traditionally used for the treatment of rheumatic and arthritic conditions. It is diuretic in action and aids the excretion of uric acid via the kidneys and is, therefore, of use in the gouty forms of arthritis. Treatment must be short-term (a few weeks only) as juniper tends to irritate the kidneys. Avoid in pregnancy.
Prepared as	Tincture, infusion (small doses).

Kumarbou
POMADERRIS ELLIPTICA

Where found	North Island of New Zealand.
Appearance	A very pretty shrub.
Part used	Herb.
Therapeutic uses	As a panacea and for the treatment of rheumatism and pulmonary disorders. Also as a blood purifier.
Prepared as	Infusion. Small doses only.

Laurel
LAURUS NOBILIS

Also known as	Bay Tree.
Where found	Europe.
Appearance	An evergreen tree with lanceolate leaves which grows up to seven or eight metres high.
Part used	Oil.
Therapeutic uses	The oil is used as a relief for rheumatism.
Prepared as	Oil for external application.

Lime Flowers
TILLIA EUROPOEA

Also known as	Linden Flowers.
Where found	Throughout Europe.

Appearance	A graceful tree.
Part used	Flowers.
Therapeutic uses	A strong but safe nervine for relief of headaches and hysteria. It is an anti-stress remedy and is often included in prescriptions to help lower high blood pressure, together with circulatory tonics.
Prepared as	Infusion.

Liquorice
GLYCYRRHIZA GLABRA

Where found	Europe and Middle East.
Appearance	A strong-growing perennial plant.
Part used	Root.
Therapeutic uses	Because of its natural sweetness liquorice is often added to medicines to improve their palatability. As a demulcent and pectoral it is particularly useful when added to cough and lung mixtures. Its soothing properties make it useful in healing internal ulcers. It is apt, however, to increase water retention and blood pressure.
Prepared as	Decoction.

Logwood
HAEMATOXYLON CAMPECHIANUM

Where found	South America.
Appearance	A massive tree.
Part used	Wood.
Therapeutic uses	To relieve diarrhoea and dysentery. Also helpful for women's disorders.
Prepared as	Decoction. Small doses.

Manaca
BRUNFELSIA HOPEANA

Where found	South America and West Indies.
Appearance	A spindly shrub.
Part used	Root.
Therapeutic uses	An alterative and for the treatment of arthritis.
Prepared as	Decoction. Small doses.

Manna
FRAXINUS ORNUS

Where found	Mediterranean countries.
Appearance	Medium-sized shrub.
Part used	Sap from cuts in bark.
Therapeutic uses	As a gentle laxative for pregnant women and as a nutritive invalid food.
Prepared as	Decoction. Small doses.

Marshmallow
ALTHAEA OFFICINALIS

Where found	Throughout Europe.
Appearance	A strong-growing herb usually found in watery places.
Parts used	Leaves and root.
Therapeutic uses	As an emollient and demulcent for incorporation in cough medicines. Also for treatment of cystitis and for soothing the alimentary canal.
Prepared as	Infusion and poultice.

Mayweed
ANTHEMIS COTULA

Also known as	Dog Fennel.
Where found	Throughout Europe.
Appearance	A low-growing herb and common weed.
Part used	Herb.
Therapeutic uses	An antispasmodic with marked tonic qualities. Excellent for migraine.
Prepared as	Infusion.

Meadowsweet
FILIPENDULA ULMARIA

Also known as	Bridewort.
Where found	UK and Europe.
Appearance	Long-stemmed herb growing almost one metre.
Part used	Herb.
Therapeutic uses	Meadowsweet, a favourite herb of Queen Elizabeth I, has a wide range of uses. Like willow bark it contains a compound from which aspirin was originally derived. The old herbalists, therefore, found it of use as a treatment in rheumatic conditions. Unlike aspirin it does not cause stomach bleeds and, indeed, it is known as the herbal bicarbonate of soda, being used for relief in cases of indigestion. As an astringent it is helpful in loose conditions of the bowel.
Prepared as	Infusion.

Motherwort
LEONURUS CARDIACA

Where found	A common garden plant in Britain and northern Europe.
Appearance	A pink-flowered shrub of handsome appearance.

Part used	Herb.
Therapeutic uses	A nervine and for the relief of menstrual symptoms. Also a tonic and stimulant and helpful for heart conditions.
Prepared as	Infusion.

Mullein
VERBASCUM THAPSUS

Where found	Throughout Europe.
Appearance	Tall perennial cylindrical plant with a tower of yellow flowers.
Part used	Leaves and flowers.
Therapeutic uses	For lung and bronchial inflammations. As an astringent, demulcent and pectoral.
Prepared as	Infusion.

Mustard, Black
BRASSICA NIGRA

Mustard, White
BRASSICA ALBA

Where found	Throughout the northern hemisphere.
Appearance	A short-growing annual herb with bright yellow flowers.
Part used	Seeds.
Therapeutic uses	A powerful irritant and emetic. For relief of rheumatic and arthritic pain.

Prepared as   Poultice.

Myrtle
MYRTUS COMMUNIS

Where found	The warmer areas of Europe.
Appearance	A strong bushy shrub.
Part used	Leaves.
Therapeutic uses	Often used as a balm for night cramp.
Prepared as	Poultice.

Night Blooming Cereus
CEREUS GRANDIFLORUS

Where found	Jamaica.
Appearance	A small branched cactus with large creamy flowers.
Part used	Plant.
Therapeutic uses	An effective heart stimulant and for relief of palpitations. Also a diuretic and helpful for prostate diseases.
Prepared as	Tincture. Use only under supervision of a medical herbalist.

Nutmeg
MYRISTICA FRAGRANS

Where found	Malaysia, Indonesia and the West Indies.

Appearance	Tall tree.
Parts used	Seeds and oil.
Therapeutic uses	Carminative, anti-emetic. Helpful in most cases of stomach upset. Can be used externally for the treatment of rheumatic pain. *Use in moderation.*
Prepared as	Powder and oil.

Oats
AVENA SATIVA

Where found	In most temperate climates.
Appearance	A common farm crop similar to wheat.
Part used	Seeds.
Therapeutic uses	An effective nerve tonic and to allay spasms. Relieves rheumatic pain.
Prepared as	Decoction. Small doses only.

Papaw
CARICA PAPAYA

Also known as	Melon Tree.
Where found	Throughout sub-tropical areas.
Appearance	A tall tree (about seven metres) with boldly serrated leaves. Only the female produces fruit.

Part used	Papain from the juice.
Therapeutic uses	As a digestive aid, helpful for duodenal and peptic ulcers.
Prepared as	Powder.

Paraguay Tea
ILEX PARAGUENSIS

Also known as	Mate Tea.
Where found	South America.
Appearance	A dense shrub.
Part used	Leaves.
Therapeutic uses	Stimulant. Very helpful in the relief of rheumatism and arthritis. Commonly used to make a pleasant tea.
Prepared as	Infusion.

Parsley
CARUM PETROSELINUM

Where found	Europe.
Appearance	Biennial umbelliferous plant with white flowers and aromatic leaves.
Parts used	Seeds, root and leaves.
Therapeutic uses	As a diuretic and in the treatment of kidney disorders, stones and gravel. Emmenagogue and in the treatment of amenorrhoea.
Prepared as	Decoction.

Parsley Piert
ALCHEMILLA ARVENSIS

Also known as	Breakstone.
Where found	Throughout Europe.
Appearance	A low-growing herb with tiny green flowers. Not related to common parsley.
Part used	Herb.
Therapeutic uses	For the relief of bladder and kidney troubles and helpful in dissolving kidney stones.
Prepared as	Infusion.

Parsley Root
PETROSELINUM CRISPUM

Where found	UK and Europe.
Appearance	Small herb.
Part used	Root.
Therapeutic uses	Carminative, diuretic, emmenagogue. Has useful anti-rheumatic properties.
Prepared as	Decoction.

Pennyroyal
MENTHA PULEGIUM

Where found	UK and Europe.
Appearance	Low-growing herb.

Parts used	Herb and oil.
Therapeutic uses	Carminative, emmenagogue, stimulant, diaphoretic. This herb has always been regarded as a reliable treatment for obstructed menstruation. Applied externally it is helpful for gout. Contraindicated in pregnancy.
Prepared as	Infusion.

Peony
PAEONIA OFFICINALIS

Where found	Southern Asia.
Appearance	Beautiful perennial that bears vivid double flowers in profusion.
Part used	Root.
Therapeutic uses	Antispasmodic and tonic.
Prepared as	Use only under supervision of a medical herbalist.

Peppermint
MENTHA PIPERITA

Also known as	Curled Mint.
Where found	Europe and North America.
Appearance	A stately herb with purple-hued stems.
Part used	Herb.
Therapeutic uses	Stomachic and carminative. Relieves sickness, flatulence and indigestion.
Prepared as	Infusion.

Pichi

FABIANA IMBRICATA

Where found	South America.
Appearance	Herb of moderate growth with tiny leaves.
Parts used	Leaves and wood.
Therapeutic uses	Hepatic. Recommended for treatment of liver disorders. Also a stimulant and diuretic and helpful for catarrhal and kidney troubles.
Prepared as	Use only under supervision of a medical herbalist.

Pipsissiwa

CHIMAPHILA UMBELLATA

Also known as	Ground Holly.
Where found	Northern hemisphere.
Appearance	A small tough shrub.
Part used	Leaves.
Therapeutic uses	As a tonic and alterative. Helpful for rheumatoid ailments.
Prepared as	Infusion.

Poke Root

PHYTOLACCA DECANDRA

Where found	North America.
Appearance	Shrub with multitude of grape-sized black berries.

Part used	Root and berries.
Therapeutic uses	For relief of rheumatism and arthritis. An emetic and cathartic. Contraindicated in pregnancy.
Prepared as	Tincture on prescription from herbalist. Small doses only.

Poplar, White
POPULUS TREMULOIDES

Where found	UK and Europe.
Appearance	Large tree.
Part used	Bark.
Therapeutic uses	Anti-rheumatic. Anti-inflammatory, antiseptic. Beneficial in all cases of muscular and arthritic rheumatism.
Prepared as	Decoction.

Prickly Ash
ZANTHOXYLUM AMERICANUM

Where found	North America.
Appearance	Medium-sized tree.
Parts used	Bark and berries.
Therapeutic uses	Diaphoretic, carminative, stimulant. Helpful for circulation disorders associated with rheumatism.
Prepared as	Tincture, tablets, decoction.

Ragwort
SENECIO JACOBAEA

Also known as	St James's Wort.
Where found	Throughout Europe.
Appearance	Erect slender herb with yellow flower.
Part used	Herb.
Therapeutic uses	For rheumatic conditions and gout. A poultice made from the herb is applied to swollen joints. An ointment can also be made and used in sciatica.
Prepared as	Poultice. Not to be taken internally.

Raspberry
RUBUS IDAEUS

Where found	Commonly cultivated in most temperate climates.
Appearance	A bush producing edible fruit.
Part used	Leaves.
Therapeutic uses	Astringent and stimulant. Useful in the treatment of painful periods, easier childbirth. The herb contains two compounds, one of which stimulates the uterus to contract during labour while the other causes it to relax. The infusion, known as raspberry leaf tea, was traditionally taken during the last few weeks of pregnancy. The infusion can also be used as

a gargle for sore throats and as a
lotion for ulcerated skin.

Prepared as   Infusion.

Red Sage
SALVIA OFFICINALIS

Also known as	Sage.
Where found	Europe and North America.
Appearance	A small herb.
Part used	Leaves.
Therapeutic uses	The plant is astringent, antiseptic, and oestrogenic. The infusion is used as a gargle for sore throats, quinsy and laryngitis. An ointment is used for painful muscles and joints. The oestrogen-like effect makes it useful as a remedy during the menopause, but it should not be taken in large doses or during pregnancy.
Prepared as	Infusion, ointment.

Rest Harrow
OMONIS SPINOSA

Found wild	Throughout Britain.
Appearance	A common herb about 60 cm high. Prickly, with small purple flowers.
Part used	Root.
Therapeutic uses	Diuretic. Helpful for rheumatism.
Prepared as	Infusion.

St John's Wort
HYPERICUM PERFORATUM

Where found	Britain.
Appearance	Sturdy yellow-flowered herb.
Part used	Herb.
Therapeutic uses	Diuretic. Expectorant, helpful for coughs and bronchial ailments.
Prepared as	Decoction.

Samphire
CRITHMUM MARITIMUM

Also known as	Rock Samphire.
Where found	England, particularly in saline conditions.
Appearance	A small herb that prefers shelter of rocks.
Part used	Herb.
Therapeutic uses	Diuretic with a beneficial kidney action. Helpful for weight loss.
Prepared as	Infusion.

Sarsaparilla
SMILAX MEDICA

Where found	South America.
Appearance	Bush.
Part used	Rhizome.
Therapeutic uses	Alterative, anti-rheumatic, antiseptic. Helpful in cases of

psoriasis and other skin ailments.
Long-standing treatment for
severe rheumatism and
rheumatoid arthritis.

Prepared as   Decoction.

Savory, Summer
SATUREIA HORTENSIS

Where found	Commonly cultivated throughout the world.
Appearance	A small shrubby plant.
Part used	Herb.
Therapeutic uses	For relief of flatulence and indigestion. Also as a poultice to reduce inflammations.
Prepared as	Decoction.

Senna
CASSIA AUGUSTIFOLIA

Where found	Arabia.
Appearance	Tree of sparse growth with distinctive grey-green leaves.
Parts used	Leaves and seed case.
Therapeutic uses	A laxative. Combine with ginger, or other aromatics to prevent griping. Small doses only. Contraindicated in pregnancy.
Prepared as	Infusion.

Shepherd's Purse
CAPSELLA BURSA-PASTORIS

Where found	Everywhere.
Appearance	Small insignificant weed with little white flowers.
Part used	Herb.
Therapeutic uses	Diuretic, usually for kidney and urinary troubles. Antiscorbutic, prevents scurvy.
Prepared as	Infusion.

Slippery Elm
ULMUS FULVA

Where found	North America.
Appearance	A great tree of spreading growth.
Part used	Inner part of bark.
Therapeutic uses	As a nutritive for invalids. Also an emollient and demulcent for healing burns and skin troubles.
Prepared as	Infusion or powder.

Spearmint
MENTHA VIRIDIS

Where found	Throughout the northern hemisphere.
Appearance	Strong-growing perennial herb.
Therapeutic uses	A stimulant and carminative suitable for young and old. It is one of the common garden mints grown for culinary use. Herbalists

often add it to medicines to improve their palatability. It has many of the qualities of peppermint and thus helps to relieve flatulence and wind. It is also antispasmodic and, taken by infusion, will help to relieve abdominal pain when this is due to dietary indiscretion.

Prepared as   Infusion.

Swamp Milkweed
ASCLEPIAS INCARNATA

Where found	United States.
Appearance	Medium-sized shrub of grotesque appearance.
Parts used	Rhizome and root.
Therapeutic uses	Cathartic. Emetic. Beneficial in treatment of arthritis and stomach disorders.
Prepared as	Infusion. Small doses only.

Sweet Chestnut
CASTANEA SATIVA

Where found	UK and Europe.
Appearance	Large tree.
Part used	Leaves.

| Therapeutic uses | Astringent. Anti-rheumatic. Helpful in cases of muscular rheumatism, lumbago and fibrositis. Of specific benefit to catarrhal conditions. |
| Prepared as | Infusion. |

Sweet Sumach
RHUS AROMATICA

Where found	Canada and the United States.
Appearance	A shrub growing to about 4ft high.
Part used	Root-bark.
Therapeutic uses	Astringent and diuretic used in the treatment of incontinence in children and in the elderly.
Prepared as	Infusion.

Thuja
THUJA OCCIDENTALIS

Also known as	Tree of life, yellow cedar.
Where found	Canada and the United States.
Appearance	A coniferous tree.
Part used	Leaves.
Therapeutic uses	The infusion or tincture is used externally as a paint for the removal of small warts. The skin is painted twice a day for several weeks. The infusion may also be used externally as a lotion for eczema.
Prepared as	Infusion (as a lotion), tincture.

Thyme
THYMUS VULGARIS

Where found	Common garden plant.
Appearance	Small perennial herb with tiny leaves.
Part used	Herb.
Therapeutic uses	Antispasmodic and tonic. Contains thymol, a strong antiseptic, useful in irritable coughs and catarrh.
Prepared as	Infusion is sweetened with honey and given in tablespoonful doses.

Water Betony
SCROPHULARIA AQUATICA

Where found	United States.
Appearance	Medium-sized herb that grows beside water.
Part used	Leaves.
Therapeutic uses	Used as an ointment and poultices for skin complaints. An excellent vulnerary.
Prepared as	Poultice.

Water Dock
RUMEX AQUATICUS

Also known as	Bloodwort.
Where found	Throughout Europe.
Appearance	One of the common dock family.
Part used	Root.
Therapeutic uses	An alterative and detergent. Helps clean and strengthen gums and relieves mouth ulcers.
Prepared as	Infusion or powder.

Wild Carrot
DAUCUS CAROTA

Where found	UK and Europe.
Appearance	Small version of cultivated carrot.
Part used	Herb.
Therapeutic uses	Diuretic, carminative. Helpful in cases of cystitis, bladder infection and gout.
Prepared as	Infusion.

Wild Yam Root
DIOSCOREA VILLOSA

Also known as	Rheumatism Root, Colic Root.
Where found	North America and tropical areas.
Appearance	Tuberous plant.
Part used	Root.

Therapeutic uses   Anti-inflammatory, antispasmodic, diaphoretic. Helpful in the treatment of rheumatoid arthritis and muscular rheumatism. Leg cramps and intermittent claudication are two other conditions which can be beneficially treated.

Prepared as   Decoction.

Willow, White
SALIX ALBA

Also known as	Common Willow.
Where found	Europe.
Appearance	Tree that grows by streams and rivers.
Parts used	Bark and leaves.
Therapeutic uses	A tonic that relieves rheumatic and arthritic conditions. Also an anti-periodic.
Prepared as	Decoction.

Wintergreen
GAULTHERIA PROCUMBENS

Where found	North America.
Appearance	A small procumbent shrub.
Part used	Leaves.

Therapeutic uses	As an astringent that controls diarrhoea. Stimulant. Used as a remedy for rheumatism and as an embrocation.
Prepared as	Ointment.

Wood Sage
TEUCRIUM SCORODONIA

Also known as	Garlic Sage.
Where found	UK.
Appearance	Small herb.
Part used	Herb.
Therapeutic uses	Respiratory infections. Astringent, anti-rheumatic. This herb has been used for many years to treat respiratory infections and also rheumatic pain and stiffness.
Prepared as	Infusion. Contraindicated in pregnancy.

Yarrow
ACHILLEA MILLEFOLIUM

Also known as	Milfoil.
Where found	Britain.
Appearance	A tiny herb.
Part used	Herb.
Therapeutic uses	A stimulant and diaphoretic. Excellent for treatment of influenza and heavy chest colds. Helpful for blood purifying.
Prepared as	Infusion.

A Guide to
Herbal Suppliers

Medical herbalists practise in most towns, while health food shops should be able to assist with the more common dried herbs. Specialist requirements, though, often need specialist stockists.

The following list is by no means complete, but should be sufficient to cover most herbs mentioned in this book.

MAIL ORDER STOCKISTS

Cathay of Bournemouth Ltd
3 Wickham Road
Bournemouth
Dorset
BH7 6JX
(Free literature on request.)

Culpeper Ltd
Hadstock Road
Linton
Cambs
CB1 6NJ

MAJOR RETAIL OUTLETS

Bournemouth   Cathay of Bournemouth Ltd
3 Wickham Road
Bournemouth
Dorset
BH7 6JX

Gerard House
736 Christchurch Road
Bournemouth,
and

	31 St Thomas Street
	Lymington
	Hants
Edinburgh	Napiers of Edinburgh
	18 Bristo Place
	Edinburgh
	EH1 1EZ
London	G. Baldwin
	173 Walworth Road
	London
	SE17 1RW
	Neal's Yard Remedies
	Neal's Yard
	Covent Garden
	London
	WC2H 9DP
Ryde	The Grail
	1 The High Street
	Ryde
	Isle of Wight
	PO33 2PN

Culpeper Herbal Shops can be found in nine major towns, including three branches in London.

A directory of medical herbalists is available from the National Institute of Medical Herbalists, 9 Palace Gate, Exeter, Devon, EX1 1JA. It is advisable to consult a medical herbalist if any doubt exists about a particular condition or suggested remedy.

Glossary of Common Medical Terms

Very often when reading, or on having a medical consultation, words are used which may not be familiar. This short list will help to make some of the more common ones a little clearer.

Alterative   Any substance that can beneficially alter the condition of a patient.

Amenorrhoea   Cessation of the menstrual flow.

Anodyne   Any substance which eases pain.

Antiseptic   Any substance that prevents putrefaction.

Antispasmodic   Any substance that prevents or relieves spasms.

Anthelmintic   Any herb acting against intestinal worms.

Aperient   Any substance producing the natural evacuation of the bowels.

Aphrodisiac   Any substance that stimulates sexual functions.

Astringent Any substance which causes contraction of body tissues.

Cardiac Any condition affecting or pertaining to the heart.

Carminative Any substance that relieves pain caused by flatulence.

Cathartic Any substance that induces stimulation of bowel action; rather stronger than aperients.

Corrective Any substance that restores normal conditions.

Debility Feebleness of health.

Degenerative Deterioration or change in tissue structure.

Demulcent Any soothing medicine.

Deobstruent Any substance that frees the natural orifices of the body.

Diaphoretic Any substance inducing perspiration.

Diuretic Any substance that increases the flow of urine.

Dysmenorrhoea Excessive pain during menstruation.

Emetic	Any substance that causes vomiting.
Emmenagogue	Any drug that stimulates menstruation.
Emollient	Any substance that soothes and lubricates.
Expectorant	Any substance that helps to clear the chest of phelgm by coughing.
Haemostatic	Any substance that checks bleeding and aids the clotting of blood.
Insecticide	Any substance that is fatal to insects.
Laxative	Any substance that induces gentle, easy bowel action.
Leucorrhoea	Any mucus discharge from female genitals.
Menorrhagia	Excessive flow in menstruation.
Myalgia	Any muscular rheumatic pain.
Narcotic	Any drug that induces stupor and insensibility.
Nephritic	Any drug that affects the kidneys.
Nervine	Any substance that restores the nerves to a normal tone.

Oxytocic Any drug that contracts the uterus and hastens childbirth.

Parturient Any product used during childbirth.

Pectoral Any substance used to allay chest disorders.

Purgative A strong laxative.

Resolvent Any substance that reduces swelling.

Rubefacient Any substance that produces inflammation of the skin.

Sedative Any substance used to placate 'nerves'.

Soporific Any substance used to promote sleep.

Stimulant Any substance used to promote the reserve power of the body and produce strength and energy.

Stomachic Any substance that allays stomach disorders.

Styptic Any substance that aids the clotting of blood.

Sudorific Any substance producing heavy perspiration.

Tonic   Any substance that, if used regularly, will promote vivacity and well being.

Vermifuge   Any substance that expels worms from the body.

Vulnerary   Any substance that promotes the healing of wounds.

FURTHER READING

Other books in this Herbal Series include:

Stress and Tension
Skin Problems
Sexual Problems
Hiatus Hernia
Irritable Bowel Syndrome

*Other Foulsham books on herbal medicine edited by David
Potterton include:*

Culpeper's Colour Herbal
Medicinal Plants